T0245213

Guidelines for the Management of Acute Head Injuries

Richard Ashpole, FRCS
David G. Hardy, FRCS
Jurgen Klein, Dip IMC RCSEd

**Haigh & Hochland
Publications Ltd**

*Published by Haigh and Hochland Publications Ltd,
174a Ashley Road, Hale, Cheshire, WA15 9SF, England*

© 1996, Ashpole, Hardy and Klein

Second edition

ISBN 1-898507-30-9

British Library Cataloguing in Publication Data
*A catalogue record for this book is available from the
British Library*
Transferred to digital printing 2006
Printed in the United States of America

Contents

Glasgow Coma Scale

Eyes

Open spontaneously	4
Open to command	3
Open to pain	2
Closed	1

Motor Response

Obeys commands	6
Localizes pain	5
Normal flexion	4
Abnormal flexion	3
Extends to pain	2
No response	1

Verbal Response

Orientated	5
Disorientated	4
Inappropriate words	3
Incomprehensible sounds	2
No response	1
Total	3–15

Note: Adequate painful stimuli include:
- nail-bed pressure
- severe sternal rub
- supra-orbital pressure

To 'localize' a hand should reach towards the site of the painful stimulus in an attempt to remove it.

DEFINITIONS
Post Traumatic Amnesia (PTA)
This is the period of time **after** a head injury during which a continuous record of events is not laid down or recalled, and is manifest as an inability to remember events for a period of time after the injury. Its duration is one indicator of the severity of the head injury.

Retrograde Amnesia
This is the period of time **prior** to a head injury for which there is no recall after the injury.

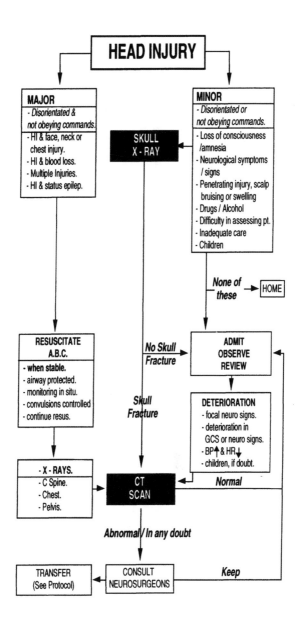

HEAD INJURY

MAJOR
- *Disorientated &*
  not obeying commands.
- HI & face, neck or
  chest injury.
- HI & blood loss.
- Multiple Injuries.
- HI & status epilep.

MINOR
- *Disorientated or*
  not obeying commands.
- Loss of consciousness
  /amnesia
- Neurological symptoms
  / signs
- Penetrating injury, scalp
  bruising or swelling
- Drugs / Alcohol
- Difficulty in assessing pt.
- Inadequate care
- Children

SKULL X - RAY

None of these → HOME

RESUSCITATE A.B.C.
- **when stable.**
- airway protected.
- monitoring in situ.
- convulsions controlled
- continue resus.

No Skull Fracture →

Skull Fracture

ADMIT OBSERVE REVIEW

DETERIORATION
- focal neuro signs.
- deterioration in
  GCS or neuro signs.
- BP↑ & HR↓
- children, if doubt.

- **X - RAYS.**
- C Spine.
- Chest.
- Pelvis.

CT SCAN

Normal

Abnormal / In any doubt

TRANSFER (See Protocol) ← **CONSULT NEUROSURGEONS**

Keep

INITIAL RESUSCITATION

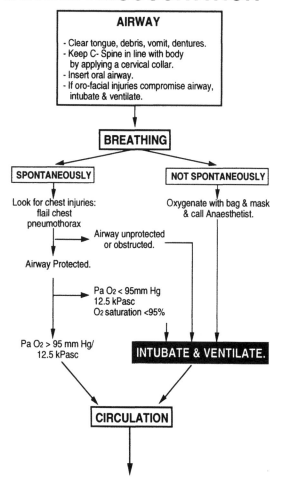

AIRWAY

- Clear tongue, debris, vomit, dentures.
- Keep C- Spine in line with body
  by applying a cervical collar.
- Insert oral airway.
- If oro-facial injuries compromise airway,
  intubate & ventilate.

BREATHING

SPONTANEOUSLY

Look for chest injuries:
flail chest
pneumothorax

Airway Protected.

Airway unprotected
or obstructed.

Pa O₂ < 95mm Hg
12.5 kPasc
O₂ saturation <95%

Pa O₂ > 95 mm Hg/
12.5 kPasc

NOT SPONTANEOUSLY

Oxygenate with bag & mask
& call Anaesthetist.

INTUBATE & VENTILATE.

CIRCULATION

Initial Resuscitation and Assessment

When a patient with a head injury arrives in the Accident and Emergency Department the first priority is assessment and support of the patient's basic life-supporting functions. This applies equally to all patients but will be more easily done in those who are essentially 'walking wounded'.

1. Assess airway

Clear the airway of a protruding tongue, debris, vomit, dentures etc. Insert an oral airway if the patient will tolerate it. Take great care of the cervical spine, which may be broken, keeping it in line with the patient's body and immobilizing it with a properly applied cervical collar, sand bags and tape as soon as is practicable. If oro-facial injuries seriously compromise the airway the patient should be intubated at this stage.

2. Assess breathing

Ascertain whether the patient is breathing spontaneously or not. If not, oxygenate with a bag and mask until an anaesthetist arrives.

If the patient is breathing spontaneously look for and treat major chest injuries e.g. pneumothorax, tension pneumothorax, flail chest and haemopneumothorax. Attach a pulse oximeter, if one is available, and aim to keep the oxygen saturation at a minimum of 95 per cent.

If the patient is **not** able to protect his airway or oxygenate himself adequately (PaO_2 > 95mmHg/12.5 kPasc and $PaCO_2$ < 40mmHg/5.3 kPasc and O_2 saturation > 95 per cent) or is vomiting then he should be intubated and ventilated by an anaesthetist.

ASSESS CIRCULATION

- Arrest obvious haemorrhage

- Measure & record heart rate & BP

- Attach monitoring for these if available

- Attach ECG & Oximeter if available

- Establish LARGE i. v. access

- Take blood for: FBC, U+E, X - match,
  Glucose, Arterial Gases.

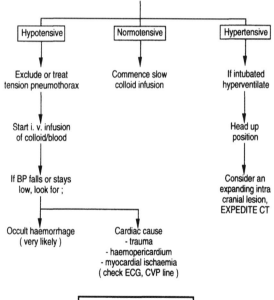

Hypotensive	Normotensive	Hypertensive
Exclude or treat tension pneumothorax	Commence slow colloid infusion	If intubated hyperventilate
Start i. v. infusion of colloid/blood		Head up position
If BP falls or stays low, look for ;		Consider an expanding intra cranial lesion, EXPEDITE CT

Occult haemorrhage (very likely)

Cardiac cause
- trauma
- haemopericardium
- myocardial ischaemia
(check ECG, CVP line)

TREAT CONVULSIONS

3. Assess circulation

The damaged brain does **not** tolerate hypotension.

Stem any major haemorrhage by applying pressure on the supplying artery. Look specifically for intraabdominal or chest injuries.

Measure and record heart rate and blood pressure, attaching appropriate monitoring equipment and also an ECG if these are available.

Establish **large** venous access and secure it meticulously.

Take venous blood samples for:
- Full blood count
- Urea and electroltes
- Glucose
- Cross - Match (make sure there's sufficient)

Take an arterial blood sample for:
- Arterial blood gases

Commence an intravenous infusion. Generally this should be of a Colloid solution (e.g. Haemaccell, Blood) in patients with a head injury. Remember that crystalloid (Dextrose or Dex/Saline) exacerbates cerebral oedema after head injury. Note that hypotension is unlikely to be due to a head injury in isolation and hypotension, hypoxia and hypercapnia all make head injuries substantially worse.

TREAT CONVULSIONS

INITIAL TREATMENT

A D U L T	
	Phenytoin
	Paraldehyde

4. Treat convulsions

Convulsions may occur following any head injury and should be treated whenever they occur, alongside any other resuscitation measures which are already taking place.

Initially convulsions should be treated with intravenous Phenytoin. It should be given slowly and titrated against the seizure activity until it is terminated. 15mg/kg is usually sufficient. For refractory fits Paraldehyde intramuscularly, 5-10mls can be used. Diazepam is best avoided because of its unpredictable tendency to cause respiratory depression.

Once the initial seizures have been controlled it is essential to commence some regular anti-convulsants, such as Phenytoin, Carbamazepine or Sodium Valproate. If Phenytoin is used its plasma level should be regularly monitored and the dose adjusted to maintain a therapeutic level (10-20 mg/l or 40-80 micromol/l).

ASSESS HEAD INJURY

- History
- Time + Mode of Injury ?
- Has patient vomited or obstructed ?

RECORD

- Glasgow Coma Score
- Localizing Signs
- Bruising
- Battle's Sign
- Lacerations
- Blood / CSF from ears , nose , mouth
- Maxillofacial injuries
- Tympanic membranes

5. Assess head injury

Many neurological disorders can be misdiagnosed as or result in a head injury and the history is often of great help. Establish time and mode of injury, and as accurate an assessment as possible of the neurological state at the scene of the injury: ask ambulance crew, police, friends or other witnesses.

Did the patient vomit at the time of the injury and therefore possibly aspirate?

Has there been any evidence of compromise to the airway?

Accurately record the initial neurological state

This consists of:

i) The Glasgow Coma Score (see accompanying chart). It is vital to record exactly what the patient can do in each category. The actual numbers and score are less important.

ii) Any localizing signs:
- Pupils, size and reaction
- Cranial nerve deficit
- Focal limb weakness

Examine the head and record details of the following using diagrams where necessary.

- Bruising
- Lacerations, including thickness and any underlying skull fractures
- Periorbital bruising /subconjunctival haemorrhage
- Battle's sign (bruising over the mastoid process)
- Discharge of blood or CSF from ears, nose or mouth
- Maxillo-facial injuries
- Tympanic membranes

FULL SYSTEMIC EXAMINATION

- Abdomen
- Pelvis
- Chest
- Limbs
- Sources of Shock

6. Carry out full systemic examination of the patient

This must include abdomen, pelvis, chest, limbs and possible sources of shock. Commence appropriate initial treatment of other injuries such as splintage, anti-tetanus prophylaxis, antibiotics and urinary catheterization. Pay particular attention to the cervical, thoracic and lumbar spine (especially if the patient is unconscious) looking for bruising, tenderness or irregularities.

7. Take a full medical history

This may have to be obtained from friends, relatives or witnesses but pay particular attention to:

- The force, nature, velocity and time of injury.
- Exact duration of any loss of consciousness.
- Any nausea and/or vomiting.
- Duration of any post-traumatic amnesia.
- Pre-existing medical conditions.
- Any fit since the injury.
- Any drugs which may have been administered.
- O_2 saturation at roadside if available.

By this stage the patient should be stabilized with an accurate assessment of all major injuries and appropriate initial treatment instigated. Attention can therefore be turned towards appropriate investigations. Many patients with more minor injuries will go through the above assessment very quickly, not requiring ventilation, splintage etc. For these patients the normal routine of history, examination and special investigations will apply.

MAJOR HEAD INJURY

• Neither orientated nor obeying commands.

X-Rays.

• Lat C-spine C1 - T1
• CXR
• Pelvis XR
• Limb + abdo as indicated
• Urgent Head CT

Major Head Injuries

All patients who are neither orientated nor obeying commands with or without other injuries.

1. Radiology
This should be performed as soon as the patient's condition allows and may be commenced in the resuscitation room using portable equipment. This should be medically supervised, especially if spinal injuries are suspected.

- Lateral cervical spine X-ray to include all seven vertebrae and the C7/T1 junction; if it is not possible to obtain or interpret these, assume an injury and leave a cervical collar in place.
- Chest X-ray.
- Pelvis X-ray.
- Limb and abdomen X-rays as indicated by the other injuries.
- Urgent head CT scan. Inform the consultant responsible for the case if he has not already been informed. In these cases of major head injury the CT is the quickest and most accurate way of assessing the intracranial compartment. Skull X-rays may be performed later in order better to define some types of injury, but at this stage there is no point in delaying a scan to obtain these.
- If immediate CT is not available then a skull X-ray may be useful. A skull fracture and altered conscious level carries approximately a one in four risk of an intracranial haematoma.

2. Assess CT scan
i) If there is any abnormality, such as swelling, air, sub or extra dural haematoma or effacement of the CSF spaces and sulci, or if in doubt, consult the regional neurosurgical unit. If transfer is recommended follow the transfer protocol outlined later in this guide.

ii) If normal, admit the patient for observation and review on the ward and continue treatment of any other injuries.

Remember that interpretation of CT scans is difficult and the surgical significance should be discussed with the neurosurgical unit.

Radiology

The following pages show X-ray and CT appearances of some of the commoner lesions seen in head injury.

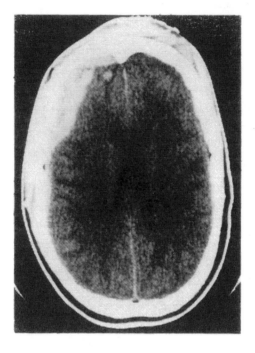

i) Right frontal acute subdural haematoma with frontal contusion and secondary mass effect

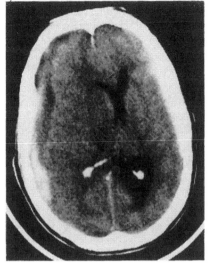

ii) Large right subdural haematoma of mixed high and low density indicating a recent bleed into a chronic subdural haematoma. There is considerable mass effect and midline shift

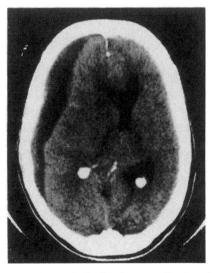

iii) Same patient as in ii, showing a recollection of low density chronic subdural fluid

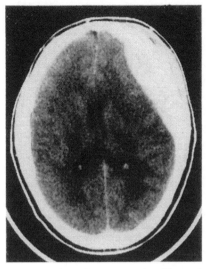

*iv) Large left frontal acute extradural haematoma
with midline shift*

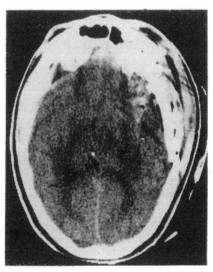

*v) Depressed fracture of a large plate of fronto-parietal
bone, with underlying left*

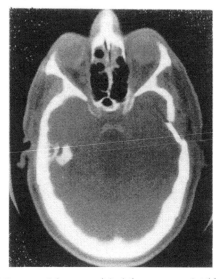

*vi) Depressed fracture of the left temporoparietal bones.
C.T. set to show bony detail*

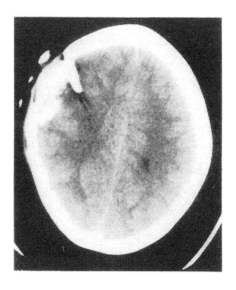

*vii) Large right frontal depressed fracture with a deeply
indriven fragment*

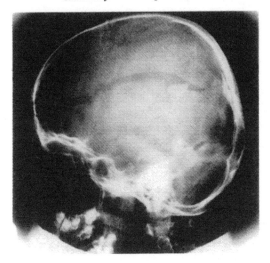

viii) Large comminuted depressed skull fracture in the parietal region with a wide fracture line extending right around the skull to the frontal region

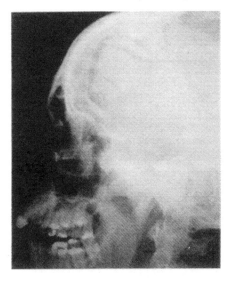

ix) Comminuted frontal bone fracture

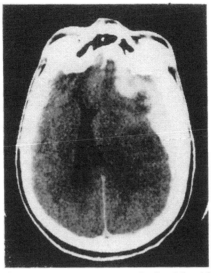

x) Extensive acute left temporoparietal subdural haematoma with mass effect, midline shift and obstructive dilatation of the right lateral ventricle

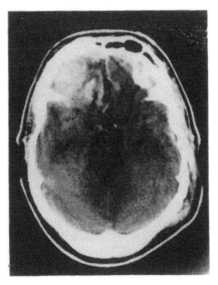

xi) Right frontal lobe contusion

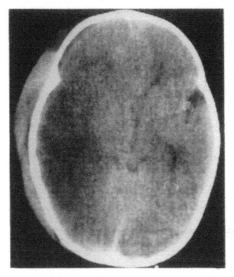

*xii) Diffuse brain swelling with obliteration of the
ventricles and midline shift*

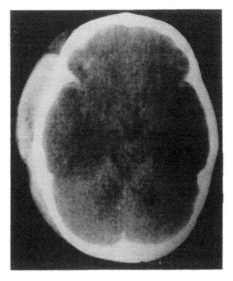

*xiii) Diffuse brain swelling with effacement of the basal
cisterns*

OBSERVATION AND REVIEW

1/2 Hourly Recordings of ;
- G.C.S.
- Pupils
- Limb movements
- Pulse
- BP
- Temperature
- Respiration

- Deteriorating G.C.S
- Worsening focal signs
- Persisting signs
- BP ↑ with HR ↓

- Urgent CT &
  Consult Neurosurgeons

Observation and Review on the Ward

This is absolutely vital as it is the sole purpose of admission for many head injuries. The sooner any deterioration is noticed the quicker corrective action can be taken.

Observations consist of half hourly recordings of:

- Glasgow Coma Scale
- Pupil reaction and size
- Limb movements
- Pulse
- Blood pressure
- Temperature
- Respiration

These must continue for at least 12 hours and each set should be complete (only exceptionally is it not possible to visualize the pupils – every effort must be made to do so). Of these signs pupillary changes tend to occur later rather than earlier.

In addition the patient should have:

i) Tetanus prophylaxis if appropriate.

ii) Flucloxacillin (or Erythromycin/Cephalosporin) if a compound or basal skull fracture exists or is suspected by the presence of blood or fluid from the nose or ears.

iii) Codeine or Paracetamol for analgesia. In patients with multiple injuries pain is often controlled with adequate splintage plus non-opioid analgesics. Opioid analgesics are usually unnecessary as in overdose they may obscure neurological deterioration. If it is necessary to give an opioid to control pain, urgent CT head scanning is vital.

iv) **No** sedation, steroids, anti-hypertensives, DDAVP or mannitol. Anti-emetics should be used sparingly because of their extra-pyramidal side effects, and their masking of important signs.

If there is any deterioration in the Glasgow Coma Scale, a worsening of any focal signs, a persistence of neurological signs beyond 12 hours or an unrelenting rise in blood pressure associated with a bradycardia the patient should be urgently re-scanned and discussed with the neurosurgical unit. Head injuries can deteriorate rapidly, even between sets of observations so any change must be acted upon.

MINOR HEAD INJURIES

• Disorientated or not obeying commands at worst.

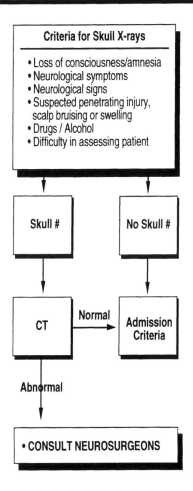

Criteria for Skull X-rays

• Loss of consciousness/amnesia
• Neurological symptoms
• Neurological signs
• Suspected penetrating injury, scalp bruising or swelling
• Drugs / Alcohol
• Difficulty in assessing patient

| Skull # | No Skull # |

| CT | Normal → | Admission Criteria |

Abnormal

• CONSULT NEUROSURGEONS

Minor Head Injuries

This group consists of those patients who at worst are either disorientated or are unable to obey commands; in other words they are only a single point short on the Glasgow Coma Scale. They may of course have other injuries.

1. Criteria for skull X-ray

Anyone satisfying any of the following nationally recommended criteria should undergo an AP, lateral and Towne's (sub-mento-vertical) skull X-rays, in addition to any X-rays indicated for other injuries.

- Loss of consciousness or amnesia at any time since the injury.

- Any neurological symptoms including headache or nausea.

- Any neurological signs, including vomiting and blood or fluid from the nose or ears, or bruising over the mastoid (Battles' sign).

- Any suspected penetrating injury or scalp bruising or swelling.

- Any other cause for a depression of conscious level such as drugs or alcohol. *(Note that if the patient is under the influence of alcohol or uncooperative, high quality X-rays may be difficult to obtain. In such circumstances it is acceptable to admit the patient for observation and review and delay the X-rays until the patient is more cooperative.)*

- Difficulty in assessing the patient, particularly children and the post-ictal.

Those with a demonstrated or suspected skull fracture, including those with evidence of a basal skull fracture such as blood or fluid from the nose, ear or mastoid bruising should proceed to CT scan and if this is abnormal neurosurgical advice should be sought. If the CT is normal they should be admitted for observation and review on the ward (see previous section). If the CT is abnormal, or if there is any difficulty in determining the surgical significance of CT findings the case should be discussed with the neurosurgeon.

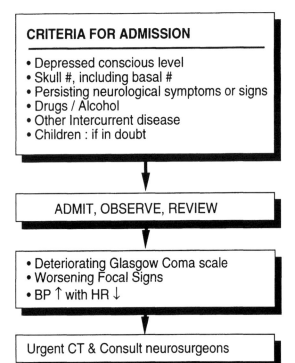

CRITERIA FOR ADMISSION

- Depressed conscious level
- Skull #, including basal #
- Persisting neurological symptoms or signs
- Drugs / Alcohol
- Other Intercurrent disease
- Children : if in doubt

ADMIT, OBSERVE, REVIEW

- Deteriorating Glasgow Coma scale
- Worsening Focal Signs
- BP ↑ with HR ↓

Urgent CT & Consult neurosurgeons

2. Criteria for admission

Anyone satisfying any of the following nationally recommended criteria should be admitted to the ward for observation and review.

- Disorientation or any other depression of conscious level at the time of examination.

- Skull fracture, including the presence of blood or fluid from the nose or ear, or bruising over the mastoid (Battle's sign) indicative of a basal skull fracture.

- Persisting neurological symptoms or signs such as headache, nausea or vomiting.

- Any other cause for a depression of conscious level such as drugs or alcohol.

- Any major intercurrent diseases e.g. haemophilia.

- Lack of a responsible adult to care for them upon their return to home.

- In the case of children if there is any doubt at all as to their fitness to be discharged.

Any of these patients who show a deterioration of their Glasgow Coma Scale, or an increase or persistence of a focal neurological deficit for more than 12 hours should be scanned and discussed with the neurosurgeons.

3. Criteria for discharge

Patients who do not fulfil any of the above criteria may be discharged home as long as there is a responsible adult to care for them. A sheet of instructions and things to look out for should be given to the responsible person (**not** to the patient; it is difficult to consult a checklist if your own consciousness is clouded). This group is quite small and consists mainly of people who may have been briefly knocked out, with minimal post-traumatic amnesia and little more than a minor headache, and who have someone at home to look after them.

Head injury advice

Any patient who does not require admission after a head injury should have a head injury advice sheet given to the person who is responsible for his immediate care, **not** to the patient himself. Some units use a card which can be dated, with one part for the patient and one part for the carer. This can be very useful for those frequent attenders at casualty departments who may amass several of these cards. The casualty officer then knows when the most recent visit occurred. The Addenbrooke's head injury advice sheet is shown below.

This patient has received a head injury. He/she has had a thorough examination and is now considered fit to return home. However, as it is not always possible to be sure that all will be well in the future, you are advised to note the instruction given below.

DO NOT TAKE ALCOHOL

If you notice any signs such as:
Increasing drowsiness
Persistent headache
Persistent nausea or vomiting
Persistent double vision

Please come to the Accident and Emergency Department immediately.
Telephone number: Cambridge (01223) 217118

Transfer Protocol

If a patient is accepted for transfer to a neurosurgical unit the following criteria must be satisfied in order to effect a safe and controlled transfer, in addition to any specific treatments that may have been necessary for head, neck and other injuries.

1. Respiration
Pa O_2 of at least 80 mmHg (10 KPasc)
Pa CO_2 no greater than 40 mmHg (5.3 KPasc)
A clear, adequate protected airway. If there is any doubt about this, the patient should be intubated and ventilated.

2. Circulation
BP greater than 100 mmHg systolic
Pulse preferably less than 100
Large iv access; blood or fluid replacement commenced.
Cross-matched blood, if available, to accompany patient.

3. Other injuries
Diagnosed.
Stable, especially neck injuries.
Adequate primary treatment begun (if a ruptured spleen or other viscus is suspected then neurosurgeons should be consulted before transfer is arranged).

4. Timing
Transfer should take place after resuscitation has been completed and the patient is stable.

5. Documentation
All notes, X-rays, and CT scans must accompany the patient.

TRANSFER PROTOCOL

- Respiration
- Circulation
- Other Injuries
- Timing
- Documentation
- Escort
- Drugs

6. Escort

Medical escort must be appropriate to the injuries sustained and if the patient is intubated then this must be an anaesthetist with appropriate resuscitation equipment and drugs. An accurate transfer chart should be kept.

7. Drugs

There is no place for steroids in the management of head injury. It may be necessary to give mannitol to effect a safe transfer but this should only be done after seeking advice from the receiving neurosugical unit.

Pharmacopoeia of Drugs used in Head Injury

These regimens and doses are guidelines for adults. Do check with the recommendation and warnings in the current edition of the BNF and take into account any other medicines that the patient may be taking at the time. For children all doses should be adjusted for weight and should be checked with a paediatrician if there is any doubt.

Carbamazepine:
Initially 100-200mg bd orally, increased to 80mg-1.2g daily in divided doses. Optimal plasma concentration 4 -12mg/1 (20-50 micromol/1)

Codeine phosphate:
30-60mg orally or intramuscularly 4 to 6 hourly

Erythromycin:
500mg qds

Flucloxacillin:
500mg qds iv via burette or orally

Mannitol:
200 mls of 20 per cent soln iv over 20 mins (adults) (may give up to 1g/kg body weight)

Metoclopramide:
10mg intramuscular, orally or iv, twice or three times daily

Paracetamol:
0.5-1g 4 to 6 hourly, orally

Paraldehyde:
5-10ml intra muscularly up to 20ml daily, 5ml /site

Phenytoin:

A loading dose of 1-1.5g in adults (15mg/kg given over half an hour if i.v); then 300 mg per day iv or orally in divided doses; then adjust dose according to blood levels. Optimal plasma concentration 10-20mg/1 (40-80 micromol/1)

Sodium valproate:

600mg-2g daily in divided doses orally; monitoring plasma levels

Sucralfate:

1g qds to the nasogastric tube or orally one hour before meals and at bedtime

Tetanus toxoid:

0.5ml stat intra-muscularly

Driving Advice

Anyone suffering a single fit or who has undergone intracranial surgery is obliged to inform the DVLA at Swansea as well as his own motor insurers. As a result of this the DVLA may require the patient to authorize the disclosure of his medical records to the centre in order to assess his fitness to drive. As a rule someone who has suffered a fit will lose his licence for an initial period of one year; and patients undergoing intracranial surgery will lose it initially for six months to a year depending on the nature of the operation. Once a patient has remained fit free for one year, depending on his circumstances, he may then reapply for a driving licence.

Rehabilitation

'Headway' is a national organization who help care for and rehabilitate head injured patients. The telephone number is given below.

Useful Telephone Numbers

DVLA	01792 772151
Headway National HQ	0115 9240800